Dr. Oleksandr Gerasymovych

MonkeyPox (MPOX): How to Treat and How to Prevent

The author, the publisher and all those who have contributed in various capacities to the publication of this work cannot guarantee that the information contained therein is accurate or complete in all its parts; furthermore, they cannot be held responsible for any errors or omissions or for the results obtained from the use of such information. Readers should therefore verify the information with other sources. In particular, they should verify the specific information that accompanies the pharmaceutical product they intend to administer to ensure that there have been no changes in the recommended doses or in the contraindications to its administration; this verification is particularly important in the case of recently introduced or rarely used drugs.

Copyright information. © Oleksandr Gerasymovych, 2024.

Abbreviations

CDC - Centers for Disease Control and Prevention

COVID-19 - Coronavirus disease 2019

DNA - Deoxyribonucleic acid

DRC - Democratic Republic of the Congo

ECDC - European Center for Disease Control and Prevention

EIS - Epidemic Intelligence Service

ELISA - enzyme-linked immunosorbent assay

FDA - U.S. Food and Drug Administration

IRF - Integrated Research Facility

MPOX - Monkey Pox Virus

MPXV - Monkey Pox Virus

NIAID - National Institute of Allergy and Infectious Diseases

PHEIC - Public health emergency of international concern

PHIL - Public Health Image Library

VARV - variola virus

WHO - World Health Organization

Index

About the author	6
Preface	8
I. Epidemiology	9
II. Etiology	15
III. Variants	22
IV. Origin of the virus	23
V. Mechanisms of transmission	25
VI. Pathophysiology	26
VII. Pathological anatomy	29
VIII. Clinical presentation	32
Symptoms and signs	32
Risk factors	39
Susceptibility to MPX Disease	39
IX. Diagnosis	43
Epidemiological data	43
Clinical data	47

Laboratory findings	47
Instrumental diagnostics	47
Differential diagnosis	48
X. Complications	49
XI. Treatment	51
XII. Prognosis	53
XIII. Prevention	54
Animals and Pets Management	59
Vaccination	61
XIV. Epilogue	65
Bibliography	68

About the author

Internal medicine doctor, graduated from Dnipro State Medical Academy in 2016, Ukraine. In 2018 I completed specialization in the city of Dnipro (in Internal Medicine). In 2012-2013 – internship in Italy (at the orthopedics and Internal medicine departments in Fabriano. On July 2021 - successful validation of the Ukrainian diploma at the University of Perugia in Italy. Author of the books "Coronavirus and arterial hypertension", "Prevention of coronavirus infection"; co-author of the books "Coronavirus and pregnancy", "Country 38 or Ukrainian anomaly", "Orthonairoviruses and Wetland virus", "Dangerous Vaping", "How to Treat Warts at Home". In 2020, I received WHO certificates "Clinical management of SARI", "Prevention and control of novel coronavirus (COVID-19) infection". In November 2020, I attended a workshop on COVID-19 in Italy: "Do we share? Coronavirus, not just a clinical challenge" with the participation of microbiologists, an infectious disease specialist, an epidemiologist, internists, an anesthetist and an economist. In November-December 2020 - volunteering at the Department of Hygiene and Prevention of the Municipality of Perugia ("Contact tracing COVID-19" project) during the COVID-19 pandemic in the Umbria region. In May 2021 - participation in the seminar "Use of COVID-19 Vaccines: Explaining Rare Thrombosis with the AstraZeneca Vaccine" in Italy. I have participated in more than 30 conferences, including: XXIV Ukrainian Congress of Heart Surgeons, VI Scientific Session of the State Institution "Institute of Gastroenterology", Ukrainian Symposium "Pain Control", etc.

What experts say about my book ["COVID-19 from A to Z"](#):

"I was amazed by the "breadth" of the work, it is a truly remarkable review"

Roberto Burioni, Professor of Virology and Microbiology, Vita-Salute San Raffaele University, Milan.

"It seems to me to be a complete and well-documented text with a copious bibliography. I will suggest it to the students"

Prof. Fabrizio Pregliasco, Health Director of the IRCCS Galeazzi Hospital – Sant'Ambrogio, Full Professor of General and Applied Hygiene in the Section of Virology of the Department of Biomedical Sciences for Health of the University of Milan.

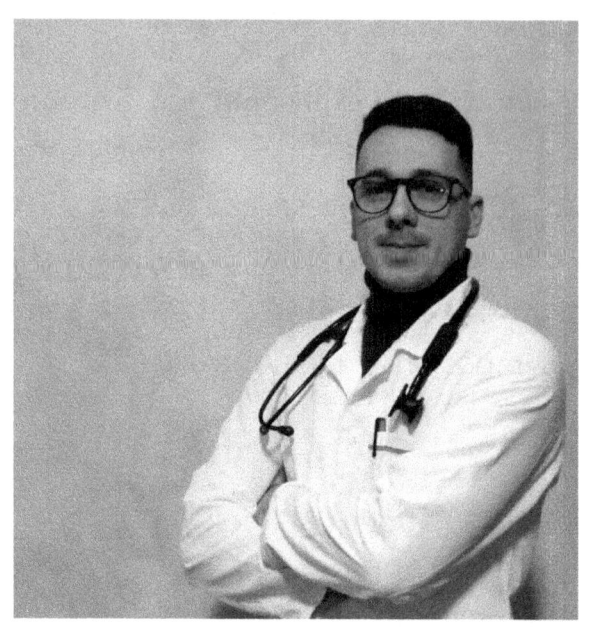

Preface

Why worry about the disease called "monkeypox"? Because the virus that causes it (smallpox virus) shares many of the characteristics of the smallpox virus (VARV). Smallpox occurs in 2 variants:

- Variola minor (mortality rate 1.2%);

- Variola major (mortality 30%-40%).[1b]

I. Epidemiology

Between 1980 and 1985, 282 cases were reported in Zaire at the time of first identification in humans. Their ages ranged from 1 month to 69 years and 90% were under 15 years old. No mortality cases were reported among vaccinated patients, while the average mortality in unvaccinated cases was 11%, with higher rates in children (15%). [5]

Recent Mpox cases [1b]:

- 2003: a small outbreak in the USA linked to illegal trafficking of African animals (< 30 cases);

- 2018: 1 case among British healthcare workers, 1 case in a traveler from Singapore;

- 2019: 1 case in a British traveler, 1 case in an Israeli traveler;

- 2021: 1 case among British travellers + 2 secondary cases infected in England; 1 case in a US traveler;

- 2022: 1 case in a US resident with no travel history.

Epidemiological situation as of 23 May 2022 (ECDC) [1b]:

• Since the disease was first identified on 7 May 2022 in the United Kingdom, a total of nine cases have been confirmed in the United Kingdom. Eight of the nine cases have no travel history and are not related to the travel-related case confirmed on 7 May.

• Since 18 May, 26 additional cases have been confirmed in Belgium (2), France (1), Italy (1), Portugal (14), Spain (7) and Sweden (1).

• Portugal has reported 20 additional suspected cases and Spain has reported 23 additional suspected cases awaiting laboratory confirmation.

The global outbreak, which began in May 2022 and has so far affected more than 27,000 people, was declared a public health emergency of international concern by the WHO on 23 July 2022. [6]

As of 23 May 2022, there were 67 confirmed cases in nine EU/EEA Member States and at least 42 other suspected cases were under investigation.

At that time, early case studies suggested descent from a common ancestor belonging to the (less severe) West African variant.[7]

Epidemiological situation as of 2024 [8]:

Europe

A total of 27,529 cases of mpox (formerly named monkeypox) have been identified through IHR mechanisms, official public sources and TESSy up to 05 July 2024, 14:00, from 46 countries and areas throughout the European Region. Since the last report, in the last three months, 349 cases have been reported from 18 countries and areas. Over the past 4 weeks, 100 cases of mpox have been identified from 10 countries and areas.

Case-based data were reported for 27,424 cases from 42 countries and areas to ECDC and the WHO Regional Office for Europe through The European Surveillance System (TESSy), up to 05 July 2024, 10:00.

Of the 27,424 cases reported in TESSy, 27,239 were laboratory confirmed. Furthermore, where sequencing was available, 500 were confirmed to belong to Clade II, formerly known as the West African clade. No cases of Clade I have been reported in the Region. The earliest known case has a specimen date of 07 March 2022 and was identified through retrospective testing of a residual sample. The earliest date of symptom onset was reported as 17 April 2022.

The majority of cases were between 31 and 40 years-old and male (98%). Of the 12,527 male cases with known sexual orientation, 97% self-identified as men who have sex with men. Among cases with known HIV status, 38% were HIV-positive. The majority of cases presented with a rash (93%) and systemic symptoms such as fever, fatigue, muscle pain, chills, or headache (69%). There were 885 cases hospitalised (7%), of which 301 cases required clinical care. Eight cases were admitted to ICU, and 10 cases of mpox were reported to have died.

USA

In the United States, case numbers peaked in early August 2022. By the end of the first year of the outbreak, more than 30,000 U.S. mpox clade II cases were reported and more than 140,000 specimens of suspected mpox were tested.[63]

Two years later, many things are different in the United States [62]:

-Clade II mpox is still circulating, but at much lower levels, mostly in small clusters in urban areas.

-We are able to quickly test for mpox at laboratories nationwide, and we have expanded monitoring for mpox in wastewater in communities across the country.

-We have an ongoing clinical trial to learn more about the effectiveness of TPOXX for treatment of mpox.

-And we have ample supplies of mpox vaccine – anyone who is eligible can get the recommended two doses.

-But some things remain the same: in the United States, clade II mpox is still mostly being spread through sexual and intimate contact, and gay, bisexual, and other men who have sex with men are at the highest risk of getting mpox.

The number of illnesses reported recently is far below the peak of the outbreak in July and August 2022, when the national 7-day average was more than 450 cases a day (or more than 11,000 per month). Between January and September 2023, there were fewer than 180 cases reported per month. In October 2023, there was an uptick to about 250 that month. Case counts have remained consistent at about 250 a month since then. [62]

In 2023, there were a total of 1,700 cases. So far in 2024, a total of 1,122 cases have been reported. [62]

A new CDC study[64] indicates that getting two doses of mpox vaccine works to prevent mpox, yet only 23% of eligible people have received the vaccine. It's very rare for people to get mpox after they've been fully vaccinated.

August 14, 2024, WHO Director-General Dr Tedros Adhanom Ghebreyesus has determined that the upsurge of mpox in the Democratic Republic of the Congo (DRC) and a growing number of countries in Africa constitutes a public health emergency of international concern (PHEIC) under the International Health Regulations (2005) (IHR). [9]

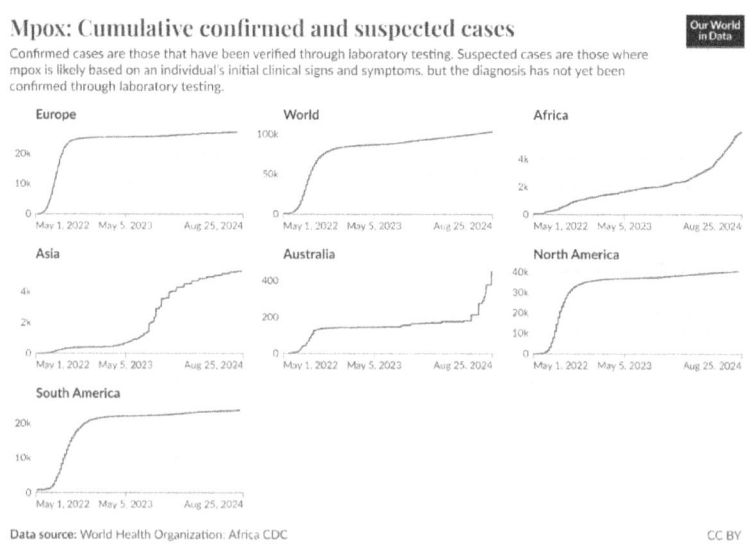

Edouard Mathieu, Fiona Spooner, Saloni Dattani, Hannah Ritchie and Max Roser (2022) - "Mpox" Published online at OurWorldInData.org. Retrieved from: 'https://ourworldindata.org/mpox' [Online Resource]

II. Etiology

Monkeypox is caused by the Monkey Pox virus.

Taxonomy of monkeypox virus (MPXV):

- Domain Acytota (i.e. virus)

- Group I (DNA viruses)

- Kingdom Varidnaviria

- Subkingdom Bamfordviridae

- Phylum Nucleocitoviricota

- Class Pokkesviricetes

- Order Chitovirales

- Family Poxviridae

- Subfamily Cordopoxvirinae

- Genus Orthopoxvirus

- Virus type Monkeypox virus.

Size: 400 x 230 nm (visible under a light microscope).

Other characteristics [1b]:

- Unconventional geometry, neither icosahedral nor "spiral" (sometimes called "brick-shaped");
- The presence of external protrusions, called "ridges".

Serological studies are not enough for laboratory diagnosis; PCR is required, including all human poxviruses. [1b]

The internal structure is also surprisingly complex. Schematically it is possible to highlight [1b]:

- External lipoprotein membrane (envelope);

- Protein nucleus (core);

- There are also two external structures or "lateral bodies" with unknown functions.

Some virological aspects [1,2,3]:

- Genome 250-300 kb

- 300 open reading frames

- From 53 to 56 virulence genes.

3 main virulence proteins of VARV[1b]:

-OP C3L complement control protein

-COP C10L IL1b antagonist protein

-COP E3L IFN resistance protein: they are deleted or fragmented in MPX.

The human smallpox virus comes from a common ancestor of rodents and camels. Smallpox virus and monkeypox virus are therefore not closely related, they share structural and biological aspects, but they are not the same virus. [4]

Monkeypox virus was named so because it was first identified in some macaques brought to Singapore from the Belgian Congo (1958). [10]

In fact, MPX is able to infect practically all primates (including humans) and practically all rodents.

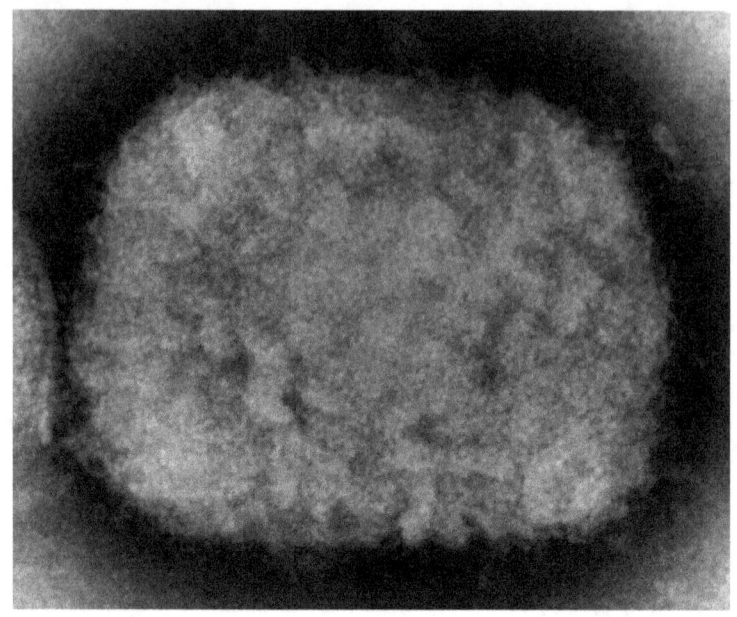

Public Health Image Library (PHIL) 22663: This electron microscopic (EM) image depicted a mpox virion, obtained from a clinical sample associated with the 2003 prairie dog outbreak. It was a negative stain image, showing a single, brick-shaped particle, covered with whorled filaments.

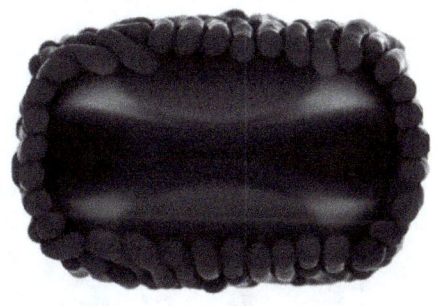

Public Health Image Library (PHIL) 26088: This illustration depicts a cut-away view of a single black-colored mpox virion on a white background, showing an interior dumbbell-shaped core, containing the DNA of the virus, and lateral bodies. These are surrounded by an exterior coat of surface filaments.

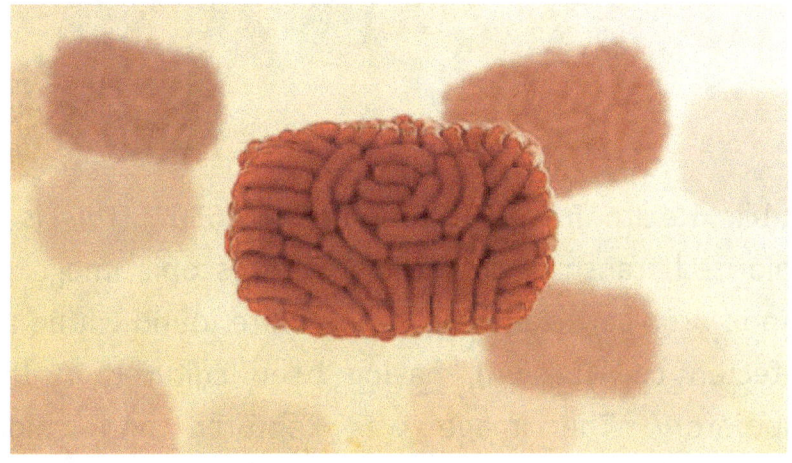

Public Health Image Library (PHIL) 26092: This illustration depicts a number of mpox virions, each with its intact exterior coat composed of surface filaments, sometimes seen in a whorled pattern.

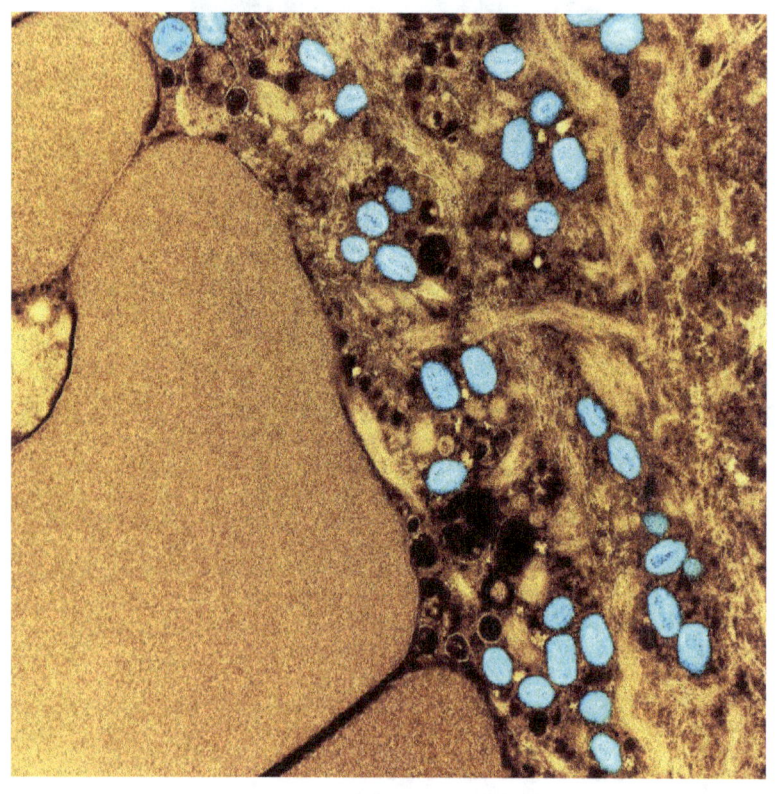

Public Health Image Library (PHIL) 26502. This is a colorized transmission electron microscopic image of mpox virus particles (teal), which were found within an infected cell (brown), having been cultured in the laboratory. The image was captured and color-enhanced at the National Institute of Allergy and

Infectious Diseases (NIAID), Integrated Research Facility (IRF), located in Fort Detrick, Maryland.

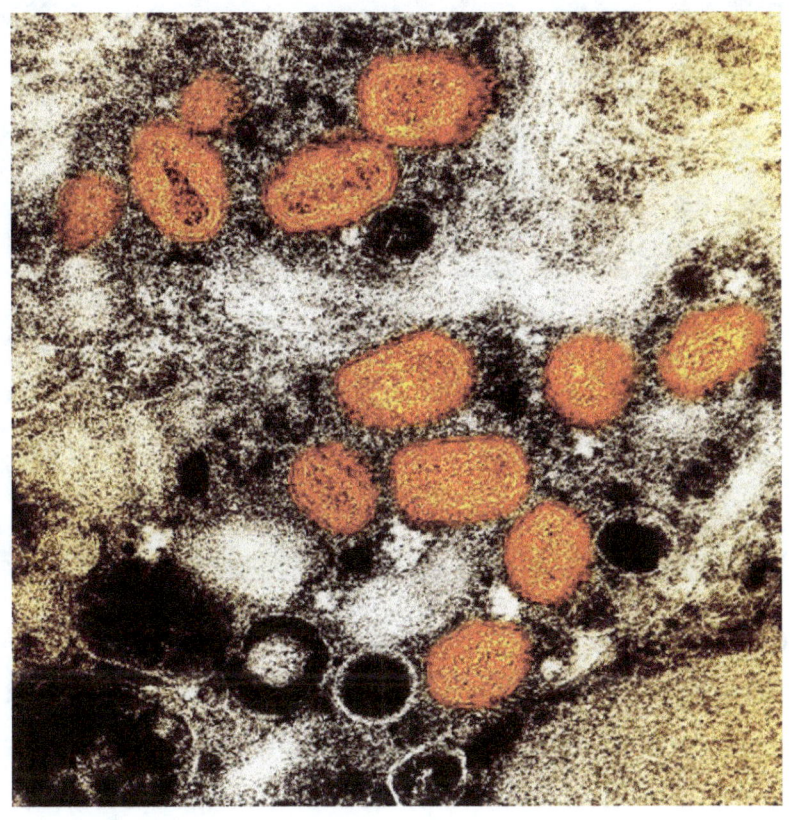

Public Health Image Library (PHIL) 26503. This is a colorized transmission electron microscopic image of mpox virus particles (orange), which were found within an infected cell (brown), having been cultured in the laboratory. The image was captured and color-enhanced at the National Institute of Allergy and Infectious Diseases (NIAID), Integrated Research Facility (IRF), located in Fort Detrick, Maryland.

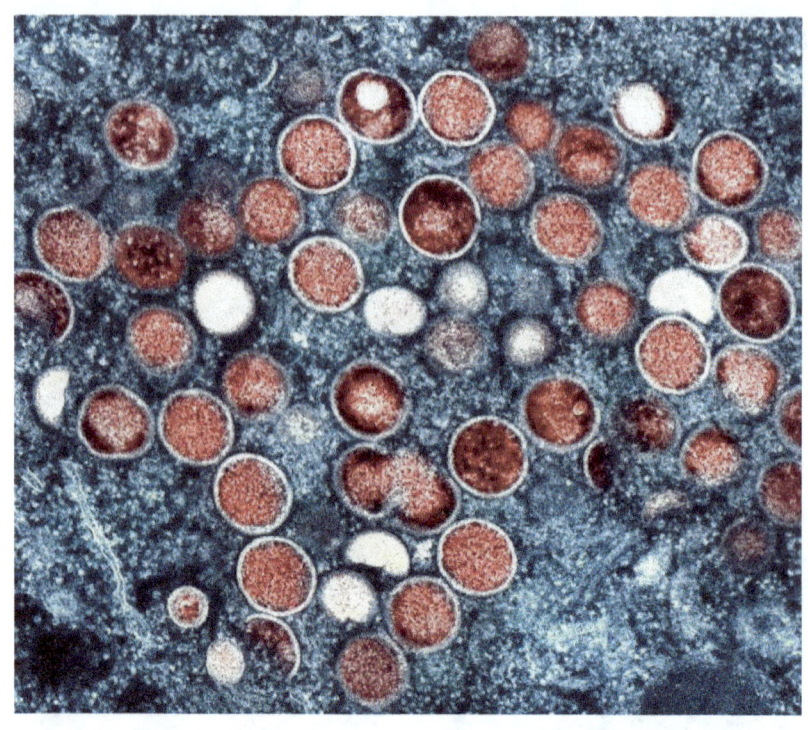

Public Health Image Library (PHIL) 26500. This is a colorized transmission electron microscopic image of mpox virus particles (red), found within an infected cell (blue), that had been cultured in the laboratory. The image was captured and color-enhanced at the National Institute of Allergy and Infectious Diseases (NIAID), Integrated Research Facility (IRF), located in Fort Detrick, Maryland.

III. Variants

MPX has been confirmed to be genetically divided into two variants:

- West African variant

- Central African variant.

The West African variant has a deletion of some pathogenic genes, which is fully expressed in the Central African variant. [11]

Genome sequencing has revealed differences between the current outbreak strains, classified as clade IIb, and the prior clade IIa and clade I viruses, but whether these differences contribute to virulence or transmission has not been determined. Clade differences in mpox virus virulence have that order: clade I > clade IIa > clade IIb. [55] It is suggested that clade IIb is evolving diminished virulence or adapting to other species. [56]

IV. Origin of the virus

The family Poxviridae consists of 22 genera and 83 species of two subfamilies: Chordopoxvirinae (18 genera and 52 species) and Entomopoxvirinae (4 genera and 31 species). [12]

The genus Orthopoxvirus affects humans and animals, with 12 identified members. The most well-known member is the variola virus, which causes smallpox; others are MPXV, vaccinia virus (smallpox vaccine virus), Abatino macacapox virus, Akhmeta virus, Camelpox virus, Cowpox virus, Ectromelia virus, Raccoonpox virus, Skunkpox virus, Taterapox virus, and Volepox virus. [12]

Two viral clades, the West African and Central African (Congo Basin) clades, have been identified. [13] The central African viruses are more virulent than the West African [14, 15]. During the 2003 U.S. outbreak, the Central African clade of human MPX disease was associated with higher morbidity, death, human-to-human transmission, and viremia. [16] The central African clade is reported to be more severe and shows a higher fatality rate (10%) than the West African clade (4%). [17, 18] The differences in virulence stem from variabilities in genome organization caused by deleted gene regions and gene fragmentation in open reading frames. [19]

Thus, sample collection from the different areas, individuals, and clades is vital for determining the genetic properties of the MPXV and confirming the cases and research facilities. [20]

V. Mechanisms of transmission

Human-to-human transmission of MPX has been documented since the 1970s. [21]

Human-to-human transmission can occur [1b]:

• Through the respiratory route,

• Through respiratory droplets,

• Through contact with contaminated surfaces,

• Through contact with biological fluids.

MPX is a DNA virus with an envelope and a protein core. This gives orthopoxviruses remarkable environmental stability and resistance to disinfection procedures. MPX is not inactivated by high/low temperatures and is highly resistant to desiccation and UV radiation. Therefore, it is estimated that it can survive [1b]:

• Up to 96 hours in the rotating chamber [22],

• Up to 56 days on surfaces [23].

Vertical transmission of monkeypox can lead to fetal infection. In a series of four pregnant women from the DRC with monkeypox, two had early abortions and one had a second-trimester fetal loss.[24] The stillborn had a generalized rash, and MPX virus was detected in fetal tissue, umbilical cord, and placenta. In particular, the most virulent strain was strain 1; the effect of strains 2/3 on the fetus is not well known.[25]

VI. Pathophysiology

The average size of the MPXV ranges between 200 and 250 nm. The MPXV replicates in the cytoplasm of the infected host cell and has a core area with lateral bodies, double-stranded deoxyribonucleic acid (dsDNA), and a lipoprotein envelope. Micropinocytosis, viral endocytosis, and cell membrane fusion facilitate viral entry via the nasopharyngeal, oropharyngeal, subcutaneous, intradermal, and intramuscular pathways. Inflammatory immune-mediated phagocytosis is triggered by MPXV replication at the inoculation, which causes MPXV to spread to the blood, lymph nodes, tonsils, bone marrow, spleen, and other organs. [53] The MPXV genome and proteins are released into host cells under the control of MPXV mature virions (MV) and enveloped virions (EV). Following MPXV mRNA transcription and translation, intracellular mature virions (IMV) with viral DNA encoding the virus are produced. IMVs wrapped in Golgi apparatus-derived membranes create intracellular enveloped virions (IEVs), which fusion with the host inner cell membrane to make cell-associated virions (CEVs) before being released into extracellular areas to form extracellular enveloped virions (EEV).[26]

MPXV has the wide-ranging effects on the immune system, from stimulation to modulation to memory, effects on the immune cells and molecules, including natural killer cells, macrophages, neutrophils, lymphocytes, cytokines, interferons, chemokines, and complement. [27]

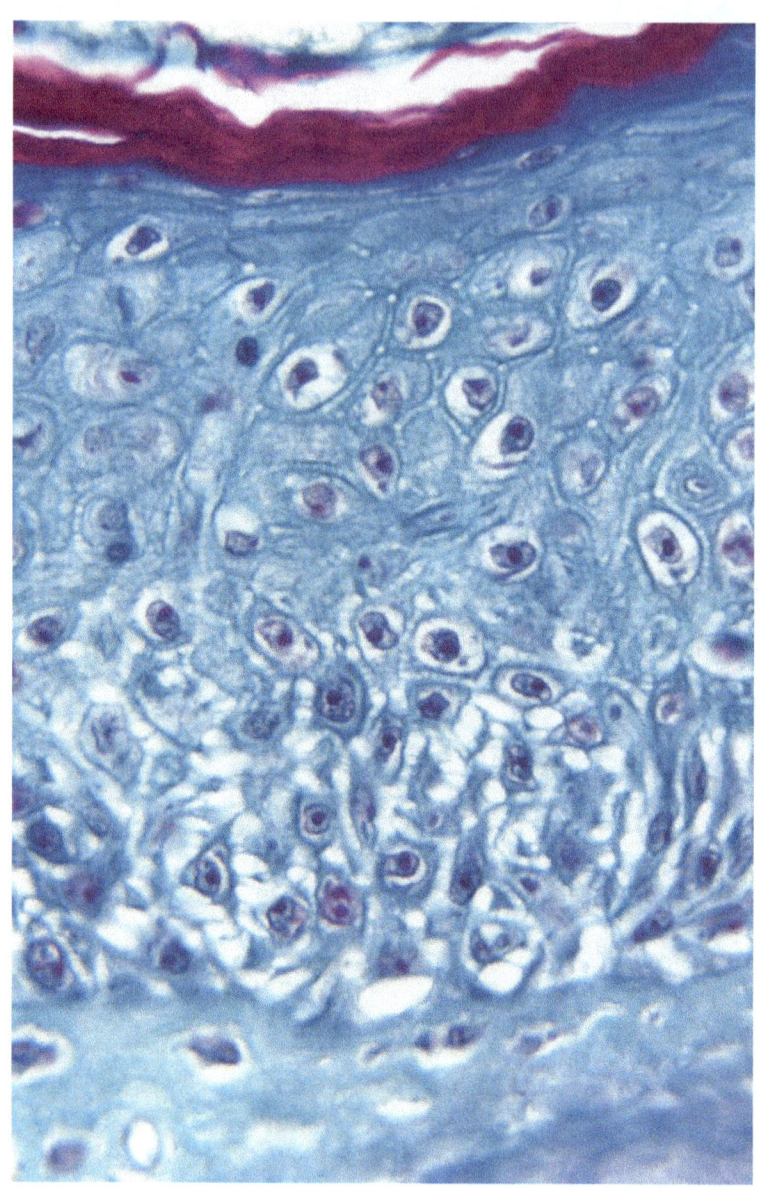

Public Health Image Library (PHIL) 21056. Under a magnification of 500X, this image depicted a section of skin tissue, harvested from a lesion on the skin of a monkey, that had been infected with mpox virus. The specimen was obtained on day-2 of the rash development.

Other images of human skin biopsy specimens are available at nejm.org/doi/full/10.1056/NEJMoa032299.

VII. Pathological anatomy

In human, the clinical progression of lesions is mirrored histologically with ballooning degeneration of basal keratinocytes and spongiosis of a mildly acanthotic epidermis progressing to full thickness necrosis of a markedly acanthotic epidermis containing few viable keratinocytes. A lichenoid-mixed inflammatory cell infiltrate is present, which exhibits progressive exocytosis with the keratinocyte necrosis. Inflammation of the superficial and deep vascular plexes, eccrine units and follicles is also present. Viral cytopathic effect is manifest by multinucleated syncytial keratinocytes. Immunohistochemically, viral antigen is detected within keratinocytes of the lesional epidermis, follicular and eccrine epithelium and few dermal mononuclear cells. Electron microscopy reveals virions at various stages of assembly within the keratinocyte cytoplasm. [28]

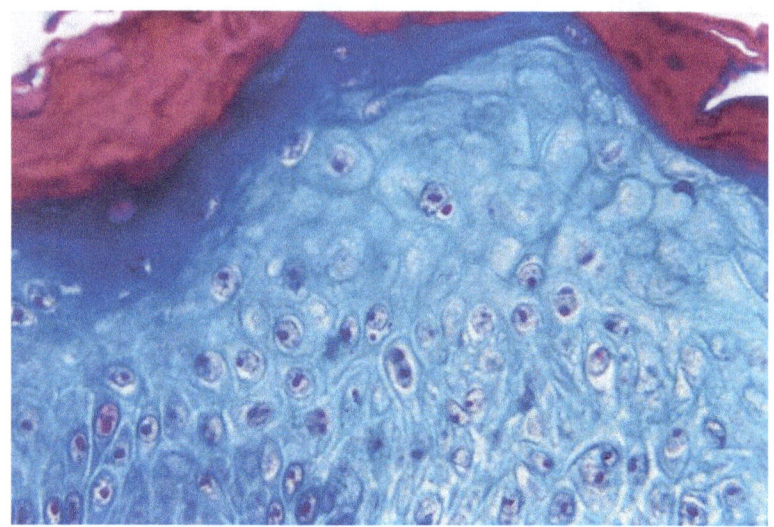

Public Health Image Library (PHIL) 21057: Under a magnification of 500X, this image depicted a section of skin tissue, harvested from a lesion on the skin of a monkey, that had been infected with mpox virus. The specimen was obtained on day-2 of the rash development.

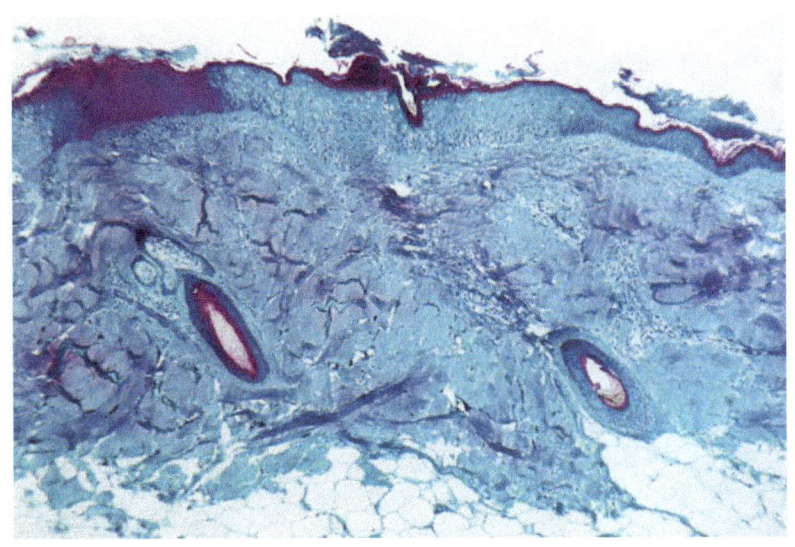

Public Health Image Library (PHIL)21069: Under a magnification of 50X, this image depicted a section of skin tissue, harvested from a lesion on the skin of a monkey, that had been infected with mpox virus. The specimen was obtained on day-2 of the rash development.

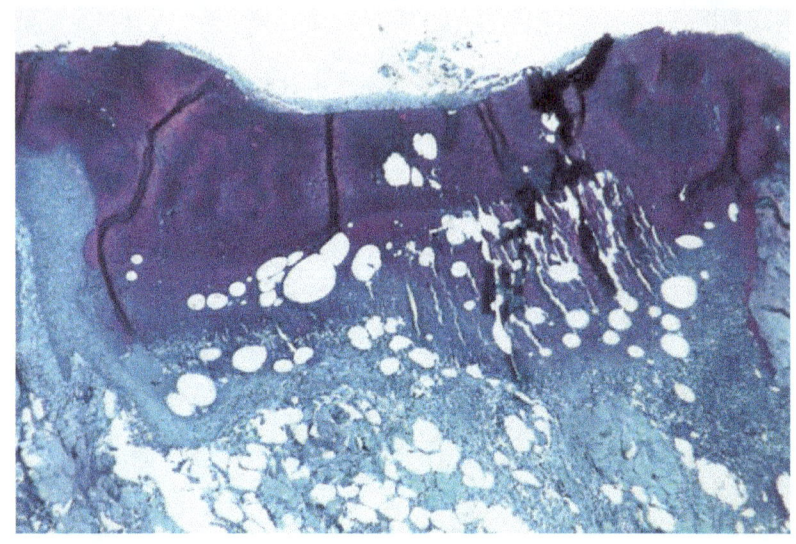

Public Health Image Library (PHIL) 21066: Under a magnification of 50X, this image depicted a section of skin tissue, harvested from a lesion on the skin of a monkey, that had been infected with mpox virus. The specimen was obtained on day-13 of the rash development.

VIII. Clinical presentation

Signs and Symptoms

MPX causes a clinical syndrome that is virtually indistinguishable from smallpox. The only difference is lymphadenopathy, which is usually absent in smallpox. After an incubation period (asymptomatic) during which the patient cannot transmit the infection, which can last from 3 to 16 days (5-21 according to some sources), a series of prodromal signs and symptoms appear. [29]

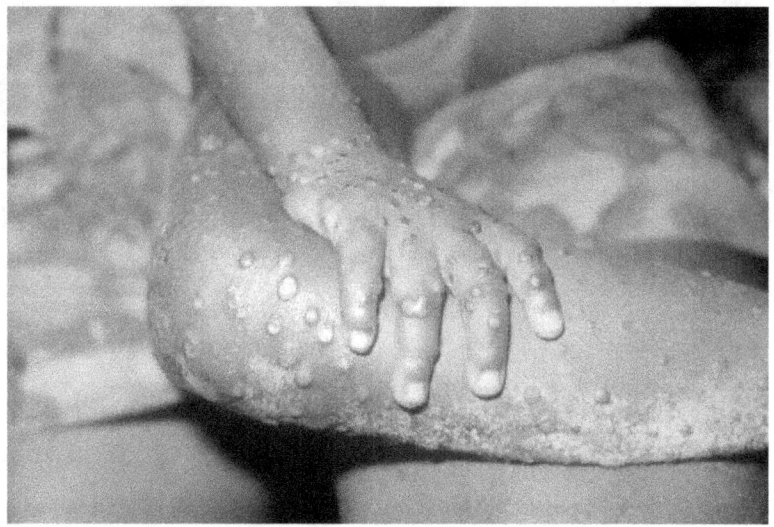

Public Health Image Library (PHIL) 2329: This image from 1971, depicts a view of the right hand and leg, of a 4 year-old female in Bondua, Grand Gedeh County, Liberia, which reveals numerous maculopapular mpox lesions, enabling you to see the similarity of these lesions to those of smallpox.

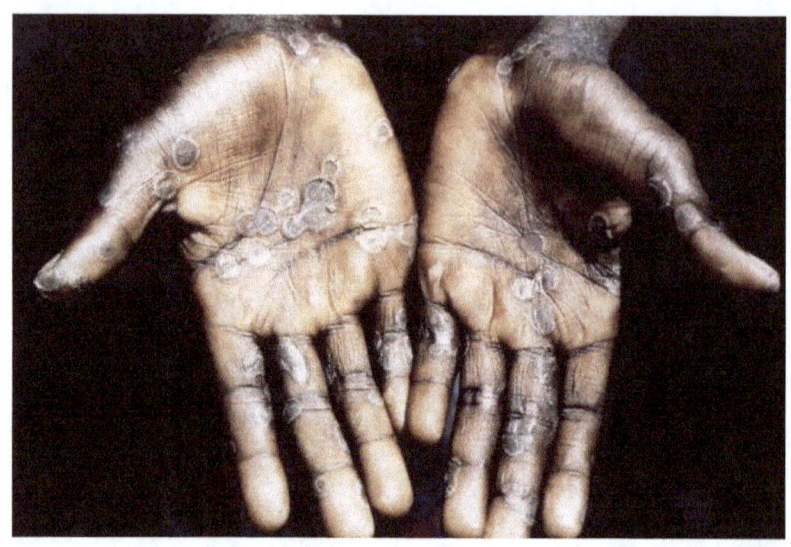

Public Health Image Library (PHIL) 12761: This 1997 image was created during an investigation into an outbreak of mpox, which took place in the Democratic Republic of the Congo (DRC), formerly Zaire, and depicts the palms of a mpox case patient from Lodja, a city located within the Katako-Kombe Health Zone, of the DRC. It is important to note, how similar this maculopapular rash appears to be when compared to the rash of smallpox, also an Orthopoxvirus.

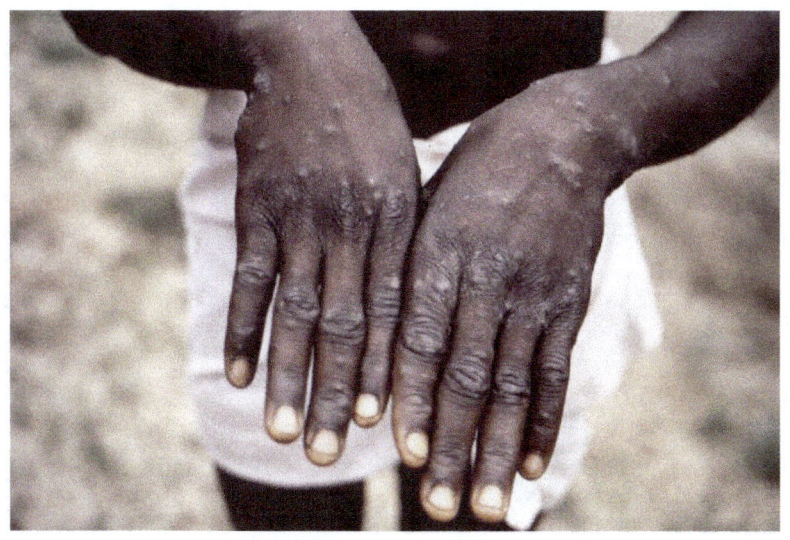

Public Health Image Library (PHIL) 12763: This 1997 image was created during an investigation into an outbreak of mpox, which took place in the Democratic Republic of the Congo (DRC), formerly Zaire, and depicts the dorsal surfaces of the hands of a mpox case patient, who was displaying the appearance of the characteristic rash during its recuperative stage. Even in its stages of healing, note how similar this rash appears to be when compared to the recuperative rash of smallpox, also an Orthopoxvirus.

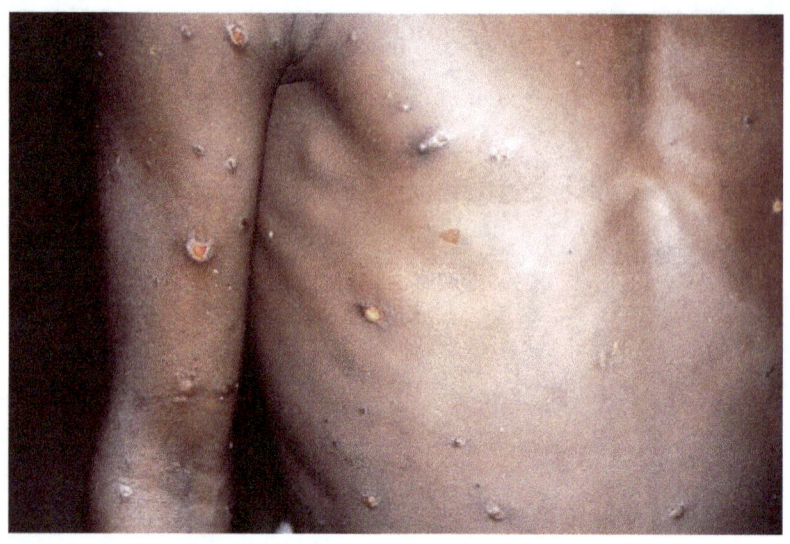

Public Health Image Library (PHIL) 12779: This 1997 image was created during an investigation into an outbreak of mpox, which took place in the Democratic Republic of the Congo (DRC), formerly Zaire. Pictured here, was the right arm and torso of a patient, whose skin displayed a number of lesions due to what had been an active case of mpox. You'll note how this rash resembles smallpox. PHIL images 12745 through 12784 depict a full slide presentation telling the story of this investigation.

After the rash appears, it has a synchronous evolutionary character.

The degree and severity of lesions varies from person to person. A rash always leaves scars.

A rash appears on the face.

Mpox lesions:

• In most cases, it begins as a rash

• Possible appearance in the form of spots

• Then it spreads to other parts of the body

• The rash has an evolutionary character:

- from a rash to a spot

- from a macule to a papule

- from a papule to a vesicle

- from a vesicle to a pustule

- from a pustule to a scarring lesion. [1b]

You can see more photos of the characteristic mpox rash at the following links (contains strong and emotional content): gov.uk/guidance/monkeypox, thelancet.com/pdfs/journals/laninf/PIIS1473-3099(22)00228-6.pdf, phil.cdc.gov/QuickSearch.aspx (enter "mpox" in the search field); thelancet.com/journals/lancet/article/PIIS0140-6736(22)01436-2/fulltext.

All MPX cases reported nonspecific and general symptoms: fever, headache, myalgia, back pain, lymphadenopathy, chills, fatigue and rash. After infection, some possible complications were evaluated such as bacterial superinfection in the affected areas, corneal infection, sepsis, dehydration, bronchopneumonia and respiratory distress. [30]

As long as the patient has active lesions on the skin, he or she can transmit the virus (i.e. until healing or crusting). [1b]

However, the first available reports suggest that this variant has specific characteristics:

- Smaller lesions, more similar in the initial phase to chickenpox;

- Lesions concentrated in the genital area in case of sexual infection;

- There may be cases (fortunately rare) without skin lesions (risk of asymptomatic carriers). [31]

Patient 1 in one study initially developed a nodular lesion at the bite site of the wrist after being bitten by a prairie dog; had developed a generalized rash during hospitalization. His condition was similar to a zoonotic infection, and his initial symptoms did not trigger the use of the smallpox detection algorithm, although he had a febrile prodrome followed by a smallpox-like rash on his extremities. After a previous case of monkeypox had been diagnosed by electron microscopy, 2 confirmatory studies were performed on biopsy specimens from this patient. [31]

Risk factors

Exposed to high risk of complications (x 10) [1b]:

- Unvaccinated subjects

- Pregnant women

- Newborns/children

- People with immunosuppression.

Susceptibility to MPX Disease

The world faces an outbreak with lots of unknowns. Factors that indicate population immunity to the genus Orthopoxvirus need to be analyzed and reported to prevent diseases involving MPX, smallpox, and the vaccinia virus. Age, sex, medical history, ethnicity, vaccination state, and possible exposure to orthopoxvirus infections indicate MPX susceptibility.[53]

The cross-protective potential of available vaccines against the Orthopoxvirus genus members is known. Since the eradication of smallpox in the 1980 s, both the vaccination status of the population and studies have slowly dropped. In 2001 a local report from Santé Publique France (the French Institute of Public Health) indicated that the smallpox vaccination rate of people born after 1979 was almost 0%, while it was 90% in those born before 1966.[32]

Seroprevalence investigation of different populations from Europe, Africa, and South America shows that all groups are vulnerable to orthopoxvirus infection; unlike uncontrolled ordinary spreading of orthopoxvirus in African countries, public immunity is also low. [32,33]

In addition, the co-infection of an HIV-positive immunosuppressed individual with MPX causes severe symptoms and a higher mortality rate. [34]

Age and vaccination status are considered susceptibility determinants. In the 2003 outbreak, an MPX history of three family members was assessed. A woman aged 30, her 33 years old husband, and her six-year-old daughter had several MPX symptoms. The man who previously received the smallpox vaccine showed mild symptoms with rashes, while the woman who was not vaccinated against MPX showed similar signs. Their child, who received all childhood vaccines except the varicella vaccine, had more severe symptoms and was hospitalized for severe encephalitis. [35]

Thus, probable protective effects of vaccination against Orthopoxvirus species and age-related immunity should be considered when considering susceptibility. [53]

In the 2022 outbreak, males, especially those having intercourse with other men, were more susceptible to transmission and showed severe symptoms. [36]

It has to be noted that lack of knowledge about how sexual transmission occurs in those people may also be the reason for the worsened outcome and thus makes these people susceptible to spreading the disease. [53]

Connection with possible animal reservoirs and suitable vectors of human transmission make individuals susceptible to MPX. [37]

Nevertheless, other potential factors of susceptibility need investigation. In addition, scientific approaches and techniques should be utilized to clarify the relationship between population genetics, viral genomics, public immunity, and disease susceptibility. Breaking down social distances and physical barriers via social events (i.e., religious meetings and sports events) or natural and man-made disasters (i.e., natural disasters and wars) expose people to infectious agents. Meanwhile, the world refugee crisis also increases spreading rate of infectious agents. At the end of 2021, 89.3 million people fled from their own country, and sought safety in other places [38], which also caused an increase in the spreading rate of viruses such as MPXV. [39]

All in all, authorities, to prevent MPXV spread should improve food aid, health, sanitation, security, camping and movement route, and housing conditions. [53]

Recently, a primary concern in FIFA World Cup 2022 was the risk of increasing the spreading rate of COVID-19 and MPX. Managing crowds is hard on its own; meanwhile, dealing with such a big hosting for the first time and the climate increases the spreading rate of infectious diseases. Dealing with all of this needs professionalism. Otherwise, both Qatar locals and people from around the globe would have been at serious risk for both MPX and other zoonotic diseases. [41]

The grouping strategy recommended by the WHO director [42] and using expertise from countries like Saudi Arabia that can manage and overcome huge crowds due to religious meetings every year could be helpful preventive activities.

IX. Diagnosis

Epidemiological data [61]

1. Suspect Case

New characteristic rash* OR

Meets one of the epidemiologic criteria and has a high clinical suspicion for mpox.

2. Probable Case

No suspicion of other recent Orthopoxvirus exposure (e.g., Vaccinia virus in ACAM2000 vaccination) AND demonstration of the presence of:

Orthopoxvirus DNA by polymerase chain reaction of a clinical specimen OR

Orthopoxvirus using immunohistochemical or electron microscopy testing methods OR

Demonstration of detectable levels of anti-orthopoxvirus IgM antibody during the period of 4 to 56 days after rash onset.

3. Confirmed Case

Demonstration of the presence of monkeypox virus (MPXV) DNA by polymerase chain reaction testing or Next-Generation sequencing of a clinical specimen OR isolation of MPXV in culture from a clinical specimen.

Epidemiologic Criteria

Within 21 days of illness onset:

Reports having contact with a person or people with a similar appearing rash or who received a diagnosis of confirmed or probable mpox OR

Had close or intimate in-person contact with individuals in a social network experiencing mpox activity, this includes men who have sex with men (MSM) who meet partners through an online website, digital application ("app"), or social event (e.g., a bar or party) OR

Traveled outside the US to a country with confirmed cases of mpox or where MPXV is endemic OR

Had contact with a dead or live wild animal or exotic pet that is an African endemic species or used a product derived from such animals (e.g., game meat, creams, lotions, powders, etc.).

Exclusion Criteria

A case may be excluded as a suspect, probable, or confirmed case if:

An alternative diagnosis can fully explain the illness OR

An individual with symptoms consistent with mpox does not develop a rash within 5 days of illness onset OR

A case where high-quality specimens do not demonstrate the presence of Orthopoxvirus or MPXV or antibodies to orthopoxvirus.

Interim Case Definitions for Clade I Mpox As of June 10, 2024 [61]:

1. Suspect Case, Clade I

Probable or confirmed mpox as defined above AND

At least one of the Clade I Epidemiologic Criteria (below)

2. Probable Case, Clade I

Probable or confirmed mpox as defined above AND

At least one of the Clade I Epidemiologic Criteria (below) AND

Clade I and clade II MPXV-negative by polymerase chain reaction testing without Next-Generation sequencing of a clinical specimen to confirm clade.

3. Confirmed Case, Clade I

Demonstration of the presence of clade I MPXV DNA by polymerase chain reaction testing or Next-Generation sequencing of a clinical specimen.

Clade I Epidemiologic Criteria

Within 21 days of illness onset:

Traveled to an area with evidence of sustained human to human transmission of clade I mpox or where clade I MPXV is endemic, OR

Reports having contact with person with confirmed, probable or suspect clade I mpox, OR

Had close or intimate in-person contact with individuals in a social network currently experiencing clade I mpox activity, OR

Had contact with a dead or live wild animal or exotic pet that is a central African endemic species or used a product derived from such animals (e.g., game meat, creams, lotions, powders, etc.).

Clinical data

The presence of a rash on the skin.

Laboratory findings

Small genomic differences between MPX and VARV lead to low reliability of currently available serological ELISA methods designed to identify VARV. A modified ELISA with an experimental target of BR129 exists, but it is not widely available. [1,2,3]

Guidelines for Collecting and Handling Specimens for Mpox Testing: https://www.cdc.gov/poxvirus/mpox/clinicians/prep-collection-specimens.html.

Instrumental diagnostics

Diagnostic samples may include:

- Skin biopsy

- Swab from skin lesions

- Swab from mucosal lesions

- Nasopharyngeal swab.

The collection of the material must be carried out as if it were a suspected SARS-CoV-2, observing all prevention rules.

Differential diagnosis

The differential diagnosis of currently identified cases is carried out with [1b]:

- Chickenpox

- Varicella zoster

- Impetigo

- Herpes simplex

- Syphilis

- Petechial typhus

- Lymphogranuloma venereum

- Molluscum contagiosum
- Measles.

The differential diagnosis is currently complicated by a series of factors [1b]:

1) little experience of healthcare workers with smallpox lesions;

2) low risk index of healthcare workers;

3) greater variability of the characteristics of the lesion based on the evolutionary stage of the pathology.

X. Complications

In most cases, the condition disappears on its own (lesions develop within 2 weeks). However, the following complications are possible [1b]:

- Bacterial superinfections
- Conjunctivitis/keratitis
- Pneumonia
- Encephalitis.

According to one study, half of all bacterial throat swabs yielded organisms compatible with clinical pharyngitis or tonsillitis. Non-toxigenic Corynebacterium diphtheriae (C diphtheriae) was isolated from a single throat swab sample in a patient with clinical tonsillitis. A single episode of bacteraemia (Escherichia coli) was detected among 49 individuals who had blood samples cultured. Antibiotic use was high in the study population with 76% (119 of 156) receiving any antibiotics during admission and 51% (79 of 156) receiving intravenous antibiotics, the majority of which were continued for more than 48 h. Individuals with clinical diagnoses of secondary bacterial infections were more likely to have lymphadenopathy, documented fever at admission, and higher early warning scores at admission. However, duration of hospital admission and results of routine blood tests were not substantially different between individuals with or without secondary bacterial infection. A single patient was admitted to a high dependency unit for monitoring during the study period and a single patient with pre-existing end-stage renal failure received renal replacement therapy as an inpatient. Two individuals were diagnosed with MPXV-associated encephalitis during hospital admission, with orthopox DNA detected in cerebrospinal fluid by PCR;

one of these two patients also developed transverse myelitis, and both recovered to their pre-admission clinical status. Five individuals had ocular complications of mpox including four with conjunctivitis, two of whom had peri-orbital cellulitis. Ten (6%) of 156 individuals required surgical procedures for complications related to MPXV infection. [40]

XI. Treatment

Although the antiviral efficacy against MPX of available drugs is unknown, they have been approved in animals against smallpox and have been used in humans. Antiviral drugs are used only in the most severe cases, for example in immunocompromised patients, in pediatrics, in pregnant and breastfeeding women, as well as in patients with lesions near the mouth, eyes and genitals. Tecovirimat (TPOXX or ST-246), brincidofovir (Tembexa or CMX001) and cidofovir (CDV, Vistide) are antiviral agents approved for smallpox. [43]

The therapeutic effect of the anti-orthopoxvirus compound ST-246 (inhibitor of the viral envelope VP37) has been evaluated in animal models, prairie dogs as pathogens of infection. ST-246 was administered intranasally to infected dogs for 14 days, starting from day zero until day three of the intranasal challenge and after the appearance of the rash. Dogs treated before the onset of symptoms were asymptomatic, while the post-rash group became ill but recovered.[44]

In another study applied to nonhuman primate models of smallpox and MPXV, ST-246 was shown to be safe, effective, and prophylactic before and after exposure to the viral agent. ST-246 is protective against disease severity and death and can be used for prophylactic or therapeutic functions.[45]

These studies have shown that human therapeutic doses of ST-246 are effective at various stages of the disease.[46]

Brincidofovir and cidofovir act as inhibitors of the viral DNA polymerase and are analogs of each other. Due to the potential toxicity to several internal organs, their use protocol is also EUA or IND. While the efficacy against MPX of cidofovir has been established in animal tests, the activity of brincidofovir has been demonstrated only for infections caused by the genus Orthopoxvirus [43].

VIG (vaccinal immunoglobulins) are hyperimmune globulins approved by the FDA to reduce the side effects of vaccination with live varicella vaccine (e.g. ACAM2000).[43]

The efficacy of VIG against smallpox and MPX has not been demonstrated. Therefore, it should be used under the IND protocol. Hyperimmune plasma collected from persons vaccinated with live vaccinia virus contains protective antibodies. In addition, insignificant antibodies against vaccinia virus with unknown immune protective functions have been detected in plasma.[47]

A safer alternative can be considered the preparation of known mixtures of monoclonal and polyclonal antibodies, which specifically recognize the epitopes of the vaccinia virus.

Host-targeting antivirals are under investigation [57]. There is currently a relevant limitation for designing drugs (i.e., the lack of solved 3D-structures of MPXV proteins) [58]. High-throughput screening and different computational methods are being used in drug discovery against mpox [58, 59]. Besides small molecules, monoclonal antibodies are currently being developed and are undergoing preclinical trials [60].

XII. Prognosis

In most cases, the disease resolves on its own (the rash develops within 2 weeks). However, complications are possible: bacterial superinfections, conjunctivitis/keratitis, pneumonia, encephalitis.

Vaccination against smallpox reduces, but does not eliminate, the risk of infection. And it appears to provide little protection from the severity of the clinical syndrome. [48,49]

XIII. Prevention

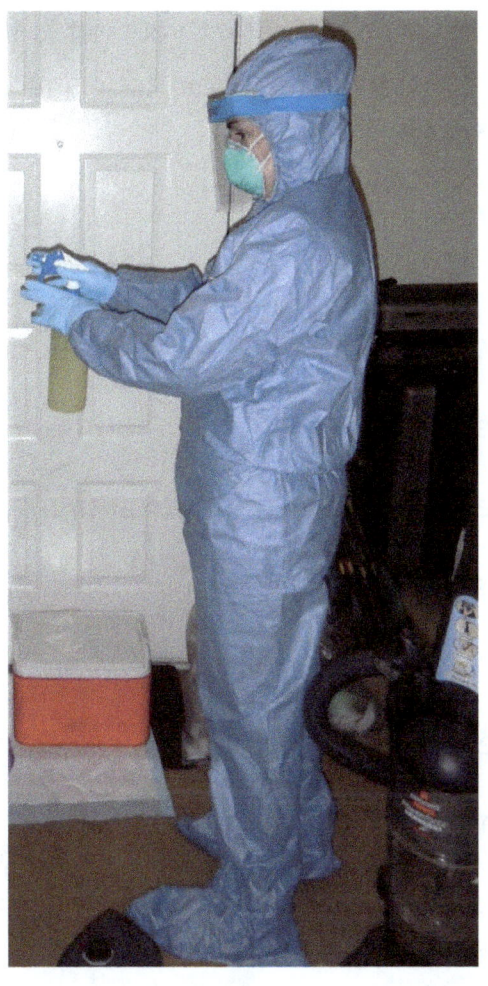

This photograph depicts Epidemic Intelligence Service (EIS) officer, Florence Whitehill (EIS Class of 2020), as she was sanitizing gloves after the collection of environmental swab samples in the residence of a patient with a mpox virus infection in Dallas, Texas, in July of 2021.

The best way to protect yourself is to follow the rules of personal hygiene, avoid touching used objects and animal waste.

Preventive measures

Each case should be considered an outbreak and managed accordingly [50]:

- Immediate reporting to local authorities

- Immediate reporting by the state authority.

The report should contain[1b]:

- Date and place of reporting;

- Name, age, sex and place of residence of the patient;

- Date of onset of first symptoms;

- Recent travel history and any information useful for contact tracing;

- Reference to impact with a probable or confirmed case;

- Tracing of close contacts and their identification (if necessary);

- Smallpox vaccination status;

- The presence of a rash;

- Presence of other clinical signs or symptoms;

- Date of confirmation or exclusion;

- Method of confirmation;

- Genomic characteristics (if available);

- Other clinical characteristics not included in the case definition, if appropriate;

- Date of hospitalization and specific certificates.

A combination of standard, contact and droplet precautions should be used in all healthcare settings if a patient presents with fever and a vesicular/pustular rash. [1b]

Due to the theoretical risk of airborne transmission of monkeypox virus, precautions should be taken whenever possible. [1b]

If monkeypox is suspected in a patient presenting to a hospital or other healthcare facility, infection control personnel should be notified immediately. [1b]

Isolate patients with suspected monkeypox in a negative-air pressure room as soon as possible. If a negative-air pressure room is not available, place patients in a private outpatient clinic. If neither option is possible, measures should be taken to minimize the impact on those around them. [1b]

These precautions may include placing a surgical mask on the patient, if acceptable to the patient, and covering any open skin lesions on the patient with a sheet or gown. [1b]

Optimal means of personal protection include [1b]:

•Use of a disposable gown and gloves for patient contact.

•Use of a NIOSH-certified N95 (or similar) filtering disposable respirator that has been tested for suitability for the healthcare worker using it, especially for prolonged contact in a hospital setting.

• Use eye protection (for example, face shields or goggles) as recommended in Standard Precautions if medical procedures may result in splashes of the patient's body fluids.

The likelihood of MPX transmission when medical personnel wear appropriate personal protective equipment (disposable gowns, disposable gloves, disposable socks or boots, respiratory protection (filtering facepiece respirator (FFP2)) and eye protection against splashes (goggles or visor) is very low, resulting in an overall low risk.

The risk for healthcare workers who have unprotected close contact with MPX cases (e.g. prolonged face-to-face contact, contact with open wounds without gloves, intubation or other invasive medical procedures) is estimated to be moderate, equivalent to close contact.

Unprotected occupational exposure in the laboratory, particularly from spills or aerosols with mucosal exposure, carries a high likelihood of infection and a moderate risk of disease (due to direct exposure of potentially significant amounts of virus to mucous membranes). The risk for unprotected laboratory personnel is assessed as high. [1b]

Animals and Pets Management[1b]

• The virus has been shown to be able to be transmitted from person to animal and from animal to person;

• There are currently no elements of risk for common domestic animals;

- However, particular attention should be paid to the risk of diffusion in the presence of rodents and other primates. It is not clear whether the virus can also infect rabbits.

During July 2022-March 2023, in one study there were collected animal and environmental swab samples within homes of confirmed human mpox case-patients and tested for MPXV and human DNA by PCR. There was also used ELISA for orthopoxvirus antibody detection. Overall, 12% (22/191) of animal and 25% (14/56) of environmental swab samples from 4 households, including samples from 4 dogs and 1 cat, were positive for MPXV DNA, but there were not detected viable MPXV or orthopoxvirus antibodies. Among MPXV PCR-positive swab samples, 82% from animals and 93% the environment amplified human DNA with a statistically significant correlation in observed cycle threshold values. These findings demonstrate likely DNA contamination from the human mpox cases. Despite the high likelihood for exposure, however, there were found no indications that pets were infected with MPXV. [54]

Recommendations for surface disinfection (recommendations of the Ministry of Health, Italy):

- Avoid dust formation;

- Avoid any activity that causes aerosol formation;

- First step cleaning with ordinary detergents;

- Second step - with sodium hypochlorite NaClO 0.1% (since household bleach has an initial concentration of 5%, dilute 1:50);

- Clean all faucets and bathroom surfaces that the patient has come into contact with;

- Use disposable cleaning products, otherwise they must be thrown away after cleaning.

Surface treatment agents recommended by the CDC: ethyl alcohol 40%, isopropyl alcohol 30%, benzalkonium chloride 100 ppm (parts per million), orthophenylphenol 0.12%, iodophor 75 ppm.

Since MPX is very resistant to high temperatures, in case of suspected or probable contamination, garments should be washed at 60°C cycles, lower temperatures will NOT inactivate the virus. [1b]

Vaccination

Since orthopoxviruses are cross-reactive, subjects vaccinated against smallpox (born before 1977) have some protection also against MPX [1b]:

- The efficacy of vaccination against smallpox is estimated at 85%.

- However, the antibody titer of smallpox gradually decreases, making revaccination necessary every ten years, which has never been done after the eradication of smallpox.

VARV has an R0 of 4 to 6. MPX has an R0 of 2 to 4. Vaccination against smallpox with an efficacy of 85% reduces the R0 of MPX to 0.95, preventing epidemic transmission. However, when the antibody coverage drops below 50%, the proliferation of MPX is no longer blocked. [51]

How vaccination was done before [1b]:

- Vaccination against smallpox took a long time because it was not done by injection.

- The vaccine was administered with a special disposable needle ("lancet"), which injected several doses of the virus under the skin, causing a small lesion.

- If the vaccination was successful, within 3-4 days a small red, inflamed lesion formed, which turned into a blister, filled with pus and began to dry out.

- In the third week after vaccination, the scab dried out and fell off, leaving a scar.

- The vaccine contained a live virus (not VARV, but vaccinia virus) that can be transmitted from a vaccinated person to their unvaccinated close contacts. The risk of side effects in case of close contact is the same as for vaccinated people.

How vaccination is done today [1b]:

- The Imvanex vaccine is administered by subcutaneous injection, preferably in the upper arm.

- In persons who have not been previously vaccinated against smallpox, two doses of 0.5 ml should be used.

- The second dose should be administered at least 28 days after the first one. [52]

Licensed vaccine products

MVA-BN was approved in 2013 for the prevention of smallpox in Canada and the European Union (EU) in persons 18 years of age and older. In 2019, MVA-BN was approved for the prevention of smallpox and mpox in adults in the United States. In the same year, Canada extended the indication of MVA-BN to mpox. On 22 July 2022, the EU approved the indication of MVA-BN for the prevention of mpox in adults. MVA-BN is not licensed for persons under 18 years of age. However, in 2022, the United States granted emergency use authorization for the use of MVA-BN in persons under 18 years of age. In Japan, LC16m8 was licensed in 1975 for smallpox without age restriction and the indication was extended for the prevention of mpox in August 2022. [65]

ACAM2000 is approved by the FDA for immunization against smallpox and is made available for use against mpox under an Expanded Access Investigational New Drug protocol. [65]

According to the manufacturer, MVA-BN is administered as a 2-dose subcutaneous injection – 0.5 mL dose containing 1×10^8 PFU (plaque forming units) – given 4 weeks apart.[65] During the global mpox outbreak, MVA-BN was also administered intradermally (0.1mL dose) in a few jurisdictions as a dose-sparing option. A systematic review[66] estimated vaccine effectiveness (VE) for a single subcutaneously-administered dose of MVA-BN at 76%. Similarly, the VE of 2 doses was estimated at 82%. The findings reveal that MVA-BN elicits a strong orthopoxvirus-specific antibody response in participants that peaks around 2 weeks after the second dose is administered, and that total orthopoxvirus-specific IgG titres and neutralizing antibody titres decline from their peak and return close to baseline levels by the 2-year mark.[67]

XIV. Epilogue

What to expect from the epidemic?

Downsides:

• Mpox is a highly spreading pathogen;

• Most of the population has weak or no antibody protection;

• The impact of the infection on a healthy but average elderly population is unknown [1b].

Upsides:

• A vaccine already exists and is effective (MVA-BN);

• Smallpox vaccines were also improved after smallpox was eradicated due to fears that the pathogen could be used as a biological weapon;

- Production lines were also designed for rapid upscaling [1b].

MPX is not new: African countries have faced MPX for a long time, with ordinary outbreaks in particular regions. Although its worldwide spreading potential is low, some regions have limitations in propagation control, prevention, and vaccination supply. However, it must be noted that there is always a possibility of an unexpected outbreak in a globalized world. MPX's spreading rate is directly correlated with the pathogenicity-dependent genetic varieties, transmission mechanism, population's lifestyle, increase in the viable host population, and changes in their habitats and vaccination profile of people. Moreover, other unknown variables also affect the spreading rate, which must be clarified further. Hence, outputs from health centers and scientific research are vital for investigating the efficacy of available vaccines on MPX. Developing a new generation of safe vaccines is essential for public and global health security. Border restrictions, developing rapid and accurate diagnostic tests, and routine screening of risk populations may prevent MPXV rotation. Determining signs and symptoms of the disease is also helpful for discriminating symbols from overlapped co-infection.

Diagnostic data accumulated in easy-to-reach applications can be used for early detection and prevention of disease. Yet the best protection method is paying attention to personal hygiene, avoiding touching used objects, and avoiding animal waste. Novel drugs and vaccines lowered the rate of diseases and thus allowed social gatherings. However, we should be aware that these diseases are still in our lives, and our decisions will shape the future and show if we made the right choice against outbreaks. [53]

Bibliography

1. Chen et al. Virology 2006;340:46-63.

1b. Monkey Pox Virus il punto della situazione al 26 Maggio 2022. Dr. Matteo Ricco'. Accessed 01/09/24.

2. Weaver et al. Immunol Rev 2008;225:96-113.

3. Shchelkunov et al. Virology 2002;297:172-194.

4. Maximum clade credibility tree for the highly conserved central genome region of the orthopoxviruses. Babkin et al. Viruses 2022;14:388.

5. Z. Jezek, M. Szczeniowski, K.M. Paluku, M. Mutombo. Human monkeypox: clinical features of 282 patients. J Infect Dis, 156 (2) (1987), pp. 293-298, 10.1093/infdis/156.2.293. PMID: 3036967.

6. Epidemia di vaiolo delle scimmie dell'OMS nel 2022: tendenze globali. https://worldhealthorg.shinyapps.io/mpx_global. Accessed: August 6 2022.

7. https://virological.org/t/first-draft-genome-sequence-of-monkeypox-virus-associated-with-the-suspected-multi-country-outbreak-may-2022-confirmed-case-in-portugal/799.

8. ECDC https://monkeypoxreport.ecdc.europa.eu (Accessed: 1.09.24).

9. WHO - WHO Director-General declares mpox outbreak a public health emergency of international concern. https://www.who.int/news/item/14-08-2024-who-director-general-declares-mpox-outbreak-a-public-health-emergency-of-international-concern.

10. von Magnus et al. Acta Pathologica Microbiologica Scandinavia, 1959, 46: 146 176.

11. Reed KD. N Engl J Med. 2004 Jan 22; 350(4):342-50.

12. International Committee on Taxonomy of Viruses, https://ictv.global/taxonomy; 2022 [accessed 8 August 2022].

13. A.M. Likos, S.A. Sammons, V.A. Olson, A.M. Frace, Y. Li, M. Olsen-Rasmussen, et al. A tale of two clades: monkeypox viruses. J Gen Virol, 86 (2005), pp. 2661-2672.

14. N. Chen, G. Li, M.K. Liszewski, J.P. Atkinson, P.B. Jahrling, Z. Feng, et al. Virulence differences between monkeypox virus isolates from West Africa and the Congo Basin Virology, 340 (2005), pp. 46-63.

15. C.L. Hutson, J.A. Abel, D.S. Carroll, V.A. Olson, Z.H. Braden, et al. Comparison of West African and Congo Basin Monkeypox Viruses in BALB/c and C57BL/6 Mice. PLOS ONE, 5 (1) (2010), Article e8912, 10.1371/journal.pone.0008912.

16. A.M. McCollum, I.K. Damon. Human monkeypox. Clin Infect Dis, 58 (2) (2014), pp. 260-267.

17. The World Health Organization (WHO). 2022 Mpox Outbreak: Global Trends. 2023. https://worldhealthorg.shinyapps.io/mpx_global/ [accessed 19 January 2023].

18. R. Sah, A. Abdelaal, A. Reda, B.E. Katamesh, E. Manirambona, H. Abdelmonem, et al. Monkeypox and its possible sexual transmission: where are we now with its evidence? Pathogens, 11 (8) (2022), p. 924.

19. J. Kaler, A. Hussain, G. Flores, S. Kheiri, D. Desrosiers. Monkeypox: a comprehensive review of transmission, pathogenesis, and manifestation. Cureus, 14 (7) (2022).

20. J.P. Thornhill, S. Barkati, S. Walmsley, J. Rockstroh, A. Antinori, L.B. Harrison, et al. Monkeypox virus infection in humans across 16 countries—April–June 2022. New Eng J Med, 387 (8) (2022), pp. 679-691.

21. Petersen et al., Infect Dis Clin N Am 2019; 33 : 1027 1043.

22. Verreault D et al. J Virol Methods, 2013; 187:333 337.

23. Wood et al. Lett Appl Microbiol 2013;57:399 404.

24. Mbala PK, Huggins JW, Riu-Rovira T, et al. Maternal and fetal outcomes among pregnant women with human monkeypox infection in the Democratic Republic of Congo. J Infect Dis. 2017;216:824–8.

25. Singhal T, Kabra SK, Lodha R. Monkeypox: A Review. Indian J Pediatr. 2022 Oct;89(10):955-960. doi: 10.1007/s12098-022-04348-0. Epub 2022 Aug 10. PMID: 35947269; PMCID: PMC9363855.

26. Paharia T., Paharia P.T. Insights into the biology of the monkeypox virus. News-Medical. 2022. https://www.news-medical.net/news/20220823/Insights-into-the-biology-of-the-monkeypox-virus.aspx. [accessed 19 January 2023].

27. Saghazadeh A, Rezaei N. Insights on Mpox virus infection immunopathogenesis. Rev Med Virol. 2023 Mar;33(2):e2426. doi: 10.1002/rmv.2426. Epub 2023 Feb 3. PMID: 36738134.

28. Bayer-Garner IB. Monkeypox virus: histologic, immunohistochemical and electron-microscopic findings. J Cutan Pathol. 2005 Jan;32(1):28-34. doi: 10.1111/j.0303-6987.2005.00254.x. PMID: 15660652.

29. Whitehouse et al. Journal of Infectious Diseases 2021;223:1870 1878.

30. J. Kaler, A. Hussain, G. Flores, S. Kheiri, D. Desrosiers. Monkeypox: a comprehensive review of transmission, pathogenesis, and manifestation. Cureus, 14 (7) (2022).

31. Lewis et al. N Engl J Med 2007;356:2112 2114.

32. L. Luciani, N. Lapidus, A. Amroun, A. Falchi, C. Souksakhone, M. Mayxay, et al. Susceptibility to monkeypox virus infection: seroprevalence of orthopoxvirus in 4 population samples; France, Bolivia Laos Mali medRxiv (2022), 10.1101/2022.07.15.2227766.

33. U.S. Food and Drug Administration (FDA). Biologics License Application (BLA) for Lynneos vaccine. 2019. https://www.fda.gov/media/131079/download. [accessed 16 September 2022].

34. A.K. Eltvedt, M. Christiansen, A. Poulsen. A case report of monkeypox in a 4-year-old boy from the DR

Congo: challenges of diagnosis and management. Case Rep Pediatr (2020), p. 8572596, 10.1155/2020/8572596.

35. J.J. Sejvar, Y. Chowdary, M. Schomogyi, J. Stevens, J. Patel, K. Karem, et al. Human monkeypox infection: a family cluster in the Midwestern United States. 190 (2004), pp. 1833-1840.

36. A. Patel, J. Bilinska, J.C.H. Tam, D.D.S. Fontoura, C.Y. Mason, A. Daunt, et al. Clinical features and novel presentations of human monkeypox in a central London centre during the 2022 outbreak: descriptive case series. BMJ, 378 (2022), Article e072410.

37. M.G. Reynolds, D.S. Carroll, K.L. Karem. Factors affecting the likelihood of monkeypox's emergence and spread in the post-smallpox era. Curr Opin Virol, 2 (2012), pp. 335-343.

38. The United Nations Refugee Agency (UNHCR). Refugee's Global report. 2022. https://www.unhcr.org/uk/figures-at-a-glance.html. [accessed 19 January 2023].

39. L. Pipito, P.D. Carlo, A. Cascio. Pustular lesions and itching in a couple of young migrants. Travel Med Infect Dis, 50 (2022), Article 102462.

40. Fink DL, Callaby H, Luintel A, Beynon W, Bond H, Lim EY, et al. Specialist and High Consequence Infectious Diseases Centres Network for Monkeypox; Dunning J. Clinical features and management of individuals admitted to hospital with monkeypox and associated complications across the UK: a retrospective cohort study. Lancet Infect Dis. 2023 May;23(5):589-597. doi: 10.1016/S1473-3099(22)00806-4. Epub 2022 Dec 22. Erratum in: Lancet Infect Dis. 2023 Apr;23(4):e121. doi: 10.1016/S1473-3099(23)00111-1. PMID: 36566771.

41. D. Subedi, S. Pantha, D. Chandran, M. Bhandari, K.P. Acharya, K. Dhama. FIFA World Cup 2022 and the Risk of Emergence of Zoonotic Diseases. J Pure Appl Microbiol, 16 (4) (2022), pp. 2246-2258, 10.22207/JPAM.16.4.47.

42. R.A. Farahat, M.O. Setti, A.Y. Benmelouka, I. Ali, T.P. Umar, et al. Monkeypox emergence and hosting a safe FIFA World Cup 2022 in Qatar: Challenges and recommendations. Int J Surg, 106 (2022), Article 106935.

43. John G. Rizk, Giuseppe Lippi, Brandon M. Henry, Donald N. Forthal, Youssef Rizk. Prevention and treatment of monkeypox. Drugs, 82 (2022), pp. 957-963, 10.1007/s40265-022-01742-y.

44. S.S. Smith, J. Self, S. Weiss, D. Carroll, Z. Braden, R.L. Regnery, W. Davidson, et al. Effective antiviral treatment of systemic orthopoxvirus disease: ST-246 treatment of prairie dogs infected with monkeypox virus. J Virol, 85 (17) (2011), pp. 9176-9187.

45. J. Huggins, A. Goff, L. Hensley, E. Mucker, J. Shamblin, C. Wlazlowski, et al. Nonhuman primates are protected from smallpox virus or monkeypox virus challenges by the antiviral drug ST-246. Antimicrob Agents Chemother, 53 (6) (2009), pp. 2620-2625.

46. Jordan Robert, Goff Arthur, Frimm Annie, L.Corrado Michael, E.Hensley Lisa, M.Byrd Chelsea, et al. ST-246 antiviral efficacy in a nonhuman primate monkeypox model: determination of the minimal effective dose and human dose justification (May) Antimicrobial agents chemotherapy, Vol. 53 (No. 5) (2009), pp. 1817-1822, 10.1128/AAC.01596-08.

47. J.W. Golden, M. Zaitseva, S. Kapnick, R.W. Fisher, M.G. Mikolajczyk, J. Ballantyne, et al. Polyclonal antibody cocktails generated using DNA vaccine technology protect in murine models of orthopoxvirus disease. Virol J, 8 (2011), p. 441, 10.1186/1743-422X-8-441.

48. Bunge et al. Plos Negl Trop Dis 2022; 16: e00110141.

49. Whitehead et al. JID 2021;223:1870 1878.

50. Ministero della Sanità - 25 maggio 2022 - 0026837-25/05/2022-DGPRE. [accessed 1 September 2024]

51. Grant et al Bull World Health Organ 2020;98:638 640.

52. EMA www.ema.europa.eu/en/documents/overview/imvanex-epar-medicine-overview_it.pdf.

53. Karagoz A, Tombuloglu H, Alsaeed M, Tombuloglu G, AlRubaish AA, Mahmoud A, Smajlović S, Ćordić S, Rabaan AA, Alsuhaimi E. Monkeypox (mpox) virus: Classification, origin, transmission, genome organization, antiviral drugs, and molecular diagnosis. J Infect Public Health. 2023 Apr;16(4):531-541. doi: 10.1016/j.jiph.2023.02.003. Epub 2023 Feb 9. PMID: 36801633; PMCID: PMC9908738.

54. Morgan CN, Wendling NM, Baird N, Kling C, Lopez L, Navarra T, Fischer G, Wynn N, Ayuk-Takor L, Darby B, Murphy J, Wofford R, Roth E, Holzbauer S, Griffith J, Ruprecht A, Harris C, Gallardo-Romero N, Doty JB. One Health Investigation into Mpox and Pets, United States.

Emerg Infect Dis. 2024 Aug 14;30(10). doi: 10.3201/eid3010.240632. Epub ahead of print. PMID: 39141926.

55. Silva, N.I.O. et al. Here, there, and everywhere: the wide host range and geographic distribution of zoonotic orthopoxviruses. Viruses. 2020; 13:43

56. Americo JL, Earl PL, Moss B. Virulence differences of mpox (monkeypox) virus clades I, IIa, and IIb.1 in a small animal model. Proc Natl Acad Sci U S A. 2023 Feb 21;120(8):e2220415120. doi: 10.1073/pnas.2220415120. Epub 2023 Feb 14. PMID: 36787354; PMCID: PMC9974501.

57. Wang, J. et al. An overview of antivirals against monkeypox virus and other orthopoxviruses. J. Med. Chem. 2023; 66:4468-4490.

58. Silva-Junior, E.F.D. The 2022 monkeypox outbreak: how the medicinal chemistry could help us? Bioorg. Med. Chem. 2022; 73, 117036.

59. Rampogu, S. et al. An overview on monkeypox virus: pathogenesis, transmission, host interaction and therapeutics. Front. Cell. Infect. Microbiol. 2023; 13, 1076251.

60. Gessain, A. et al. Monkeypox. N. Engl. J. Med. 2022; 387:1783-1793.

61. CDC - Mpox Case Definitions www.cdc.gov/poxvirus/mpox/clinicians/case-definition.html, accessed September 2, 2024.

62. CDC - Ongoing Clade II Mpox Global Outbreak https://www.cdc.gov/poxvirus/mpox/outbreak/2022-ongoing-global.html [accessed September 2, 2024].

63. The CDC Domestic Mpox Response — United States, 2022–2023 https://www.cdc.gov/mmwr/volumes/72/wr/pdfs/mm7220a2-H.pdf [accessed September 2, 2024].

64. Monkeypox Virus Infections After 2 Preexposure Doses of JYNNEOS Vaccine — United States, May 2022– May 2024. https://www.cdc.gov/mmwr/volumes/73/wr/mm7320a3.htm. [accessed September 2, 2024].

65. WHO - Weekly epidemiological record. Smallpox and mpox (orthopoxviruses) vaccine position paper. 23 AUGUST 2024, 99th YEAR. No 34, 2024, 99, 429–456. http://www.who.int/wer. Accessed 16.09.24.

66. Pischel L et al. Vaccine effectiveness of 3rd generation mpox vaccines against mpox and disease

severity: a systematic review and meta-analysis. Vaccine. 2024. doi:10.1016/j.vaccine.2024.06.021.

67. Priyamvada L et al. Serological responses to the MVA-based JYNNEOS monkeypox vaccine in a cohort of participants from the Democratic Republic of Congo. Vaccine. 2022;40:7321–7.

www.ingramcontent.com/pod-product-compliance
Lightning Source LLC
Chambersburg PA
CBHW070209230526
45471CB00002B/887